The Anti-Grind

A GUIDE TO HUMAN HEALTH OPTIMIZATION

Nick Kirk

ISBN-13: 978-0692627174
ISBN-10: 0692627170

DEDICATION

"If your actions inspire others to dream more, do more and become more, you are a leader." -John Quincy Adams

This book, as well as anything I have ever accomplished is dedicated to the people who have supported me, taught me, and inspired me the most in my life. My parents, who taught me to overcome adversity even in the most challenging of times, that attitude is everything, and most importantly to never give up on something you believe in, especially yourself.

To my Father, Tony, thank you for teaching me how to keep an open mind, and to always seek more knowledge. The pursuit to better ourselves is what will set us apart from the rest.

To my Mother, Jessica, who used to fill up grocery bags with canned goods to do exercises in the kitchen when I was a child, who has always emphasized importance on nutrition and holistic health, and who got me started on my health journey and inspired me to help others.

CONTENTS

INTRODUCTION

We've heard them all before. "Grind or go home." "Embrace the Grind." "Rise & Grind." These terms have mainly been used in the fitness community, as of late, but speak to a general mentality of working extremely hard to achieve your goals on a daily basis. This, of course, is a great mentality to have if you want to be successful, no matter what your goals may be.

The problem seems to be that people tend to take it a little too literally. They will over-train, and over-work themselves day in and day out. Over time, this can affect their long-term health in several ways. Lingering stress, inflammation, and tightness can lead to long term and permanent ailments of all sorts. Some wont show up for years later as a result of neglecting the signals our bodies are giving us.

Why focus so hard on progress with getting serious about recovery? Think of your body as a race car; you can't get out on the track and go over 100 mph everyday without having regular maintenance done on your car.

Often, we relate our mental awareness and self esteem with our physical looks, rather than how good we actually feel. We expect our physical fitness to be a representation of how happy we are.

Injuries and sickness can occur in our bodies long before we feel the affects. If preventative practices are not taken, small issues can lead to big problems that will take much longer to remedy.

We often overlook the fact that just as our physical improvements can have both positive and negative effects on our self-esteem and mental outlook, the mind can have an even more incredible influence on the body. When we are in a good state of mind, our bodies will respond quite positively.

Many options are available to you for fitness, and diet plans but there are few plans for recovery and maximum performance as it pertains to making sure your body is working at 100% of its capacity. Whether it be cross-fit, fitness competitions, martial arts, contact sports, or if you're someone who has a physically demanding, or repetitive job, you need to take good care of your body in order for it to take care of you.

We task our bodies with taking incredible amounts of stress, but we do little to give it relief, even when it takes good care of us. We often wait until our bodies break down to take action. Our bodies can take our punishment for years before giving out on us. It's important that long before issues arise, we are proactive about our preventative practices.

You can make miles of progress in your training, but if your body is performing at anything less than 100% of its capabilities, then you are doing yourself a disservice and your efforts were wasted.

I have been a wrestler since the age of 14 and after retiring from competition embarked on a professional Mixed Martial Arts career, which I am currently pursuing. I have had neck and back issues since I was a teenager, and have always had what I would consider tightly wound muscles, mostly because I've been pushing my bodies' limits for years, and have rarely done much besides taking time off in terms of real recovery.

Since surpassing the age of 30 years old, which is considered aging in the fighting world, recovery has become more and more important to me with the hope of not only extending my career professionally, but to also help counteract some of the strain I put myself through. When my career is over, and I have reached advanced age, I may actually be able to retain flexibility, range of motion, strength, endurance, health, and mental sharpness if I take care of myself along the way.

In this book, I outline some options that I have found through my own personal experiences that you can apply to your daily regimen and maximize your overall bodily health.

I want you to live healthy for longer. If you're an athlete who competes, I want you to be able to compete a little longer. If you're an average working person, then our goal is for you to get to an advanced age in life and still feel young, still have flexibility, and still have healthy muscles and joints. I want to help you avoid common illness as well as disorders and disease.

I will cover some basic info on changes you can make to your daily routines, and then add some extra things you can do to aid recovery, and balance yourself out a little bit more.

It is important to note that everyone is different. I do believe that each of these tips can help every single person, but ultimately it will be up to you to decide what works best for you.

For athletes, making a commitment to the long-term health of your body is no different than committing to work out everyday, or to read everyday, or committing to a diet. It is no different than making an investment in your retirement. Why save for retirement if you aren't preparing yourself to fully enjoy it? It is an investment in yourself that could potentially pay off in spades, saving you time and money in future medical bills and avoided injuries and sickness.

I have tried everything in this book personally. I have seen different levels of success with each of them. Everything has its place. The more you learn about your body, the more you'll learn about taking the best care of it and why it's so important.

My goal is that you'll feel better each day, and your body will operate more efficiently and comfortably. As always, in the health & nutrition communities, the knowledge is out there and is constantly growing. Keep your eyes open for new things, take advantage of the resources available to you, and listen closely to what your body is telling you.

Draw on your own experiences, learn from them, and keep an open mind. Making the choice to take care of your body can increase your quality of life by leaps and bounds. It most certainly has for me. Thank you for letting me share in my experiences with you. May you live long, healthy, and fulfilling lives.

-Nicholas Kirk

THE FOUNTAIN OF YOUTH

There are many different diet plans available to consumers. This is not a diet plan. I will, however, make the statement that you are at an increased risk of disease, sickness, and injury if you're overweight or eating an unhealthy diet.

Regardless of your diet and exercise routine, my number one suggestion to anyone looking to improve their life is to increase their water intake. The vast majority of us are not getting enough water.

Many unhealthy alternatives are presented to us, but the best thing you can do for your overall health and functionality is drink more water. One to two gallons of water should be consumed per day depending on your size. If you do not consume much water you could notice significant improvements in your skin, your weight, energy levels, and regularity.

For the athletes out there, if you just feel sluggish,

or a bit stuck in the mud you may be dehydrated. Dehydration can also have very negative effects on your brain function. This is why many of us, as children, were advised to drink a glass of water first thing in the morning.

We can easily become mildly dehydrated overnight when we sleep, and that glass of water gives our brain the energizing shot of hydration it needs for optimal functionality. Side affects of dehydration can be loss of energy, lethargy, headache, short temper, and loss of mental focus.

If you think you may be dehydrated, take in some water, and try to replenish your electrolytes if you have participated in heavy exercise.

Now, if I have successfully made my point about water, let's take this one step further. Let's add a ½-1 whole lemon squeezed into your morning water, and again in the afternoon or evening depending on your size.

Lemon water is very rich in benefits to the body. It's vital to do this in the morning on an empty stomach to receive the benefits. I have another glass of water with lemon before bed.

Lemons are rich in important vitamins and minerals like B complex vitamins, iron, magnesium, potassium, fiber, calcium, and vitamin C.

Lemon water supports brain and nerve function, heart health, boosts your immune system, stimulates your liver and detoxifies your body, reduces inflammation, balances the bodies pH levels, has a rejuvenating effect on our skin, and so much more!

I tend to spring for organic lemons, personally, as some believe they can be more potent in nutrients, and avoid being heavily sprayed with pesticides. Conventional lemons will certainly do if that's all that is at your disposal. Pink or red grapefruit juice pairs well with lemon, and has many great benefits in its own right, for those of you who want to take this step to the max. Grapefruit juice has cancer fighting antioxidants as well as a large helping of vitamins similar to that of lemon.

In as little as two weeks, for some, physical differences can be seen. This is a lifelong healthy practice that can benefit *everyone*, not just those of us who are active. Think of this as the fuel and the lubricant for the machine that you're building your life with every single day. Your digestion will improve, and will boost your bodies' ability to absorb nutrients through your food.

YOU ARE WHAT YOU EAT

Now that we have covered our daily fluid intake, let's cover your food.

As I stated earlier, fresh, raw foods are always recommended. Raw foods contain enzymes that can help aid in your bodies ability to digest and handle toxins from cooked and processed food. Get several healthy servings of vegetables into your diet. You will not be sorry in the long run.

If you have the space, and a little time to get started, I would suggest starting a small organic garden. Growing your own fruits and vegetables not only saves you money, but it gives you a sense of pride and responsibility to eat the great foods you've grown. After a little time to get it started, it doesn't take a lot to keep a garden running.

Even if you don't have space, you can grow many of the herbs we will cover in this section indoors in pots, or in a small indoor garden. You can even keep a small lemon tree if you wish. Getting creative and interactive with these things can help keep you motivated to eat healthier and will give your brain more daily reminders about being healthy, and what your overall health goals are. This will combat the "out of site out of mind" mentality.

Rather than lay out a generic diet plan that is not specific to you as an individual, or give you a list of recipes that you may or may not actually try, I would like to make a few suggestions on the seasonings that you could use in your food.

The things you season your food with can become the ace up your sleeve. You can derive a lot of valuable nutrients out of what you decide to use as your seasonings of choice.

For sweet dishes, or breakfast dishes I would recommend Cinnamon, Coconut Oil, and Honey. Cinnamon contains high levels of Manganese and fiber, and can aid in your bodies natural response to insulin. Honey is one of my personal favorites; it can do so many things for us, and is so naturally delicious it is impossible not to love!

Make sure you buy Raw Organic Honey. Honey is a powerhouse when it comes to maximizing athletic performance. Honey is superior in maintaining glycogen (energy) levels and improving recovery.

Honey carries Antibacterial and Antifungal properties, as well as Probiotic and bares special antioxidants known as flavonoids, which can help fight against heart disease and cancer. Honey can be added to your morning lemon water to help soothe irritation in your throat and help fight sicknesses and infections.

Coconut Oil is abundant in MCT's or Medium Chain Tri-glcyceride. The most important of these MCT's is Lauric-Acid, which is helpful in assisting our bodies to fight against harmful viruses and bacteria. These MCT's are also one of the most efficient sources for energy that we can put into our bodies. It will aid in a healthy metabolism, and help you burn fat. It helps to boost brain function and can be used topically on hair and skin.

For your daily meals   we will venture into more options. Our main spices we will want to work into our diet will be Himalayan Sea Salt, Oregano, Turmeric, Garlic, Sage, Rosemary, Saffron, Parsley, and Peppers. Typically it is very important to buy organic, and from trusted sources or brands when purchasing your spices as they can be highly refined and can be raised with use of pesticides.

Spices are one area in which I will advise spending the extra money, as spices generally last awhile. I will give you a short breakdown of each spice and what I love about it.

Each person's health, and taste will determine which of these are available and in what quantities.

Salt. This is the go-to seasoning for most of us when making our meals. Some diet plans suggest that you limit your salt intake. For me, its much more important **which** salt I am putting into my body.

The traditional white iodized table salt that we

are used to seeing is going to flavor your food, but really isn't going to do much else good for you. White table salt is man made, highly refined and stripped of all of its valuable nutrients. It has been linked to many current diseases and health deficiencies many people struggle with today. This is why Iodine is added after production.

Sea Salt has emerged as the healthy alternative, but which should you choose? I always recommend Himalayan Sea Salt. It has a pink hue because it still bares all of the 84 trace minerals and electrolytes that are naturally occurring, including iodine. These 84 elements work in synergy with one another to aid our bodies in countless ways. Himalayan salt is mined from 250 million year old deposits on the sea floor that were covered by lava and protected from modern pollution making it the purest salt on earth.

Oregano is a great spice to add a lot of flavor to your food. A teaspoon of oregano contains as many antioxidants as three cups of spinach. It is also a good source of fiber and vitamin K. Oregano also has antibacterial properties. This is beneficial as it can help fight against infections in your body.

Turmeric is rich in Curcumin, which is packed full of antioxidants, is known to have substantial anti-inflammatory properties, and can help manage a host of diseases ranging from rheumatoid arthritis to heart disease or even Alzheimer's. It is also a good source of Manganese and Iron.

Garlic is another important spice to keep in your diet consistently. Garlic holds many anti-inflammatory properties, and supports heart health. It is packed full of valuable flavonoids, which as we know, can help fight certain cancers. Garlic is also known to support healthy blood vessels, and blood flow as well as helping to fight the common cold.

Sage can be very tasty in the right meal and its benefits are currently being explored. Early studies show that it may protect acetylcholine in the brain, a chemical that is highly responsible in our learning capabilities.

Rosemary can actually clean your meat and rid it of cancer causing substances that can form if your meat is cooked certain ways. It also possesses a strong flavor and can enhance your meal with just a small amount.

Saffron is a wonderful herb to season meat with. It has been known around the world as a natural mood enhancer. It is loaded with antioxidants such as lycopene, as well as alpha carotene and beta-carotene.

Parsley is a delicious spice that adds a lot of color and eye appeal to your meals. Studies show that parsley is full of flavonoids, the healthy compound which has great anti-cancerous properties, and supports healthy digestion.

Peppers can be a very nutritional part of your diet. They can add a lot of spice and flavor to your meal. There are many varieties. Peppers can act as a natural thermo-genic, speeding up your metabolism and aiding in burning of fat, as well as triggering your body's natural cooling response. They are rich in vitamin c and antioxidants such as beta- carotene. As well as nutrients like manganese, iron, magnesium, and potassium. The list of health benefits is long when it comes to peppers, so I would suggest keeping them as a mainstay in your daily diet.

Adding tea to your diet can be a small addition that has a major affect on your health. The two most-healthy teas, in my opinion, are Organic Black Tea and Organic Green Tea. Both of these teas are made from the same shrub, *Camellia-Sinensis*, but with different processing methods. Black tea tends to have more caffeine.

Tea is loaded with antioxidants that treat a wide variety of issues from cancer to heart disease, promotes bone health, and supports mood. Tea can also improve brain function, as well as physical athletic performance. Tea can promote weight loss and help us burn more calories throughout that day.

Replacing your morning coffee or energy drink with tea can be a small change that has a major impact on your life. It's a great healthy way to start each morning.

This is also a great opportunity to add lemon and/or honey, which as we discussed earlier can also boast many benefits to us. Some teas can come with lemon, honey, blueberry, etc. added to it. Do your research and make sure you're getting a reliable brand of tea. You will get what you pay for with these items.

POWDERS, PILLS, AND PROTEINS

In terms of supplementation, people tend to be in one of two schools. Either you take supplements to increase your physical performance, or you don't believe in them at all.

The issue with a lot of supplement companies is that's its hard to know who to trust. There are a lot of misleading and down right fake supplement companies who are selling products that cannot do what they claim and in many instances don't contain what they claim.

Even with some reputable companies, a rising issue seems to be the chemical and synthetic compounds added to the supplements to make them taste better. I suggest doing your research, and being careful on the brands you choose as well as the supplements. Look for Certified Organic and GMO Free labels when choosing supplements.

It's important to remember that everyone is different, we are different sizes, different body compositions, our bodies break down nutrients at different rates and in different amount. There is a suggested serving size on the nutrition labels of supplements and foods that are based on an "average person," but in reality each person needs a different combination and dosage in order to achieve optimal function. Synergy is very important here.

If you have the means, it's always a good idea to have your blood tested. There are companies that can make a vitamin plan based on your deficiencies and level hormone balances. This is an excellent way to find out exactly what dosages and specifically which vitamins you need to supplement.

Some supplements that I would recommend are Vitamin D3, Oil of Oregano, Fish Oil, Multivitamin, and systemic enzyme supplements.

Vitamin D3 is a vitamin that many people today tend to be deficient in. D3 has been shown to help our bodies inhibit cancer cells, fight high blood pressure, and help with calcium uptake, which can be particularly important for women. The list of benefits is currently still growing, as well as the emphasis for supplementing this vitamin.

Oil of oregano is a good natural probiotic. Oil of oregano will reduce the amount of bad bacteria in your stomach, which helps to boost the immune system.

I advise a systemic enzyme supplement like Wobenzym-N which helps to support the body's natural inflammation response. This is not only good for overall immune support, but also for great for joints and tissues in the body.

Fish Oil, or Krill Oil are fantastic, the benefits can include better heart health, support in inhibition of cancerous cells in the body, eye and skin health, and anti-anxiety.

A good multivitamin is important. I tend to go for the natural plant based vitamins if possible. For women I would recommend a Vitamin high in folic acid and iron.

REST TO BE YOUR BEST

It's always important to get a good night's rest. The common phrase for so many of us is, "there just aren't enough hours in the day". If you have children or are busy with work or school, then finding the time for proper rest can be difficult. Motivation to find rest is often what is lacking because people just don't seem to know what a difference rest can make in the long run.

Most of our bodies' recovery and rebuilding happens when we sleep, however, there is so much more that happens. Studies show that the first four hours of a deep sleep is when the majority of our human growth hormone is produced. Human Growth Hormone is essential to our overall health. In the second half of our deep sleep our Testosterone production kicks in. Testosterone balances control so many things for us, including our moods, ability to focus, and to physically perform at our peak levels.

Sleep is where your body recovers and replenishes. It's when your brain re-organizes your memories and saves data it has taken, which boosts creativity and learning abilities. Studies show that not just physical performance, but also mental performance is stronger after a good night's rest. Sleep effects everything from our ability to fight off disease and sickness, to our overall mood, and quality of life.

It is best to sleep at slightly cooler temperatures if able. Try not to bundle up too warm when going to sleep. Sleeping at slightly cooler temperatures can boost your metabolism and help you burn fat, as well as help your body's natural ability to fight inflammation.

Inflammation, of course, has been linked to a myriad of health problems many people face today. You may have to tinker with your sleeping temperature a little if you have trouble sleeping, or if you fall asleep and wake up repeatedly throughout the night, and have difficulty going back to sleep. Studies show that the wrong temperature can be the culprit in restless nights.

Our goal here is to get the deepest sleep possible for 7-9 hours per night in order to maximize your recovery. Our bodies will take care of the rest. You need to make this a priority, as the benefits of sleep can promote you overall health, mental focus, physical performance, lifespan, and hormone production.

The detriments of a lack of deep sleep can severely inhibit all of your body's progress. You can work hard for progress and lose a lot of it by wearing your body down. I cannot stress the importance of a good night's rest enough. It could be the single best thing you do for yourself. If you absolutely cannot get this amount of sleep each night, do your best and refer to the meditation section of this guide, as its importance will become even greater for you.

REACH FOR THE STARS

Now that we have covered a couple of the basics that everyone should follow, we can get into a few things to enhance these benefits and take things a step further.

For those of us who are active and already have good practices when it comes to sleep, hydration, and our diet, we may be wondering what else can we do. Well, if you're young, and feeling great or you're not so young but not quite feeling the effects of aging, the focus becomes how to prolong this, and avoid injury or setbacks. The number one thing to emphasis, I would say, is warm your body up each day, and if possible cool it down. You can incorporate this into your workouts if you choose, if not then try to take the time each day to give yourself a good warm-up.

Yoga is a fantastic gift to give your body. If yoga classes are available to you, this is an excellent way to work on stretching, detoxifying, and positioning your body into the proper alignment. If you cannot make it to yoga classes, then I would suggest "Flow Yoga Sequence" yoga sequence series, which is authored by Sam Sarahbi, and can be purchased on Amazon or Barnes & Noble for a reasonable price.

"Flow Yoga Sequence" is a written yoga sequence that can be done in the privacy of your own home, at your own pace.

"Flow Yoga Sequence" graduates from beginner to expert. If you need help with certain poses I would suggest using your resources, go online, type in a specific pose and locate a video to help guide you.

It is important to obey the cues of the poses; don't cheat in order to do it better, it's ultimately about achieving the greater benefit. Yoga is incredibly beneficial for health. If you're an athlete, an active person, or someone who has physical issues due to work or injury, yoga could absolutely be for you. High contact athletes or those who carry a lot of stress could have immense improvements in their lives from practicing yoga.

You will practice flexibility, which we all could use, as well as balance training, strength training, core strength training, and breath control. You will get a soothing meditative relaxation and a deep detoxification. Yoga will help you sweat, which can help flush the sodium from your system and help you slim down almost immediately. It's important to replenish water and electrolytes often when practicing yoga.

If yoga just doesn't seem to be your thing, get yourself a daily stretching routine that you can do when you wake up, and then towards the end of your day as well if possible. This can allow your body to function with more fluidity, and will cause less inflammation build up; and the degeneration of joints, muscles, tendons and ligaments. It will allow your spine and hips to move into the correct alignment and will help you avoid injury due to muscle tightness.

Daily stretching can be like the fountain of youth, which can keep your body feeling young deeper into your life and is a significant investment in your future.

When stretching, if you're having any problem areas where you seem to be particularly tightly wound, I would suggest purchasing a yoga block or two and use a yoga strap or a towel to assist you with your stretches.

Keeping proper form when doing poses and stretches is crucial to achieving our goal of greater flexibility, better balance, and maximized performance. Don't break form to get deeper into stretches as it will give a false sense of progress. Proper form may seem to give slower results, however, in the long run it is exponentially more effective.

Flexibility can ease the stress that builds up in our muscles and can expel toxins from them. If you do strength training, or perform in athletics, flexibility can often translate into more power, as range of motion can play a vital role in assisting you in performing at your highest level all the time, with far less concern about personal injury.

For the average working person who doesn't engage in athletics regularly, stretching is what will fight against the bad habits we develop, like leaning forward and looking down at smart phones and computer screens, walking and sitting with improper posture for long periods of time, and neglecting our aches and pains.

If you have specific problem areas, focus on those, however its important to note that just because you aren't feeling pain, it doesn't mean everything is fine. You can have tight muscles, and if you allow them to be tight, it could be a missed opportunity to avoid injury down the road. One way or another, stretching out on a regular basis is vastly important to maintaining proper function for as long as possible.

When stretching, I suggest you set yourself a series of stretches, write it down, and time them. I use a boxing timer app that I downloaded on my smart phone. I set 25 second rounds, with 5-7 seconds in between rounds. This allows for 20-25 seconds of stretching with 5-10 seconds to switch positions comfortably. Remember to breathe through your stretches, and relax into them.

If you do not plan to stretch a second time during the day, I would add 10-15 seconds to your stretching time. Then relax into stretches and pause for half of the round, take a breath, then try to get a bit deeper if possible and relax into stretch again for remainder of round.

Take it slow and easy. Do not try to rush, and stay

true to form. You may feel sore after the first few days; this is normal and you can continue to stretch through. You should never push to the point of pain.

Warming your body up, and cooling it down goes hand in hand with stretching. Our bodies are a little more like a powerful diesel then a drag racing car. Starting cold and going 0-60, while possible, isn't doing your body any favors. You're putting unnecessary wear and tear on your body, from your joints to your organs, as well as your brain.

Taking 5-10 minutes to warm your body up in the morning before your early stretch can help increase your flexibility and speed up your progress, as well as guard against injury.

If you're someone who is active in athletics or weight/endurance training, in which you're pushing your body, you are doing your body an extreme disservice by not getting the proper warm up and cool down.

Your body will overcompensate for issues you cannot notice. When this happens, from a mechanical standpoint, you can put yourself on a path to injury.

Many injuries start long before you start feeling the pain. You must be proactive if you want to have optimal results. If you avoid a cool down, which is more common, you are causing your muscles to tighten up, and allow lactic acid to build up, curbing your progress.

Cool downs are a great time to get a second stretch in, and get the blood flowing through your muscles and tendons. Stretching will help to heal your muscles and get them on the path to recovery immediately after your workout.

Great exercises for warm ups and cool downs can be jumping rope, air-dyne bikes, jogging or a high paced walk, yoga sequences and stretching.

There are products that can aid us, such a Ben-gay, Icy-Hot, Bio-Freeze, Tiger Balm etc. I come from combat sports, in which liniment oil is the most common product used.

The products that warm tend to be the most beneficial, in my opinion. They will bring heat and blood flow to the surface and to your muscles. As you start to sweat and your pores open up, the products can get deeper into your pores and continue to warm you up further. Be careful when using products like this as to not get them close to your eyes or other sensitive areas of your bodies.

"To keep the body in good health is a duty…..otherwise we shall not be able to keep our mind free and clear." - Buddha

MIND, BODY, SPIRIT.

Meditation is an ancient form of healing that doesn't get much attention these days, especially in the realms of athletics and business. Healing and supporting your mind can be even more important than your body, in some cases.

There are many different forms and approaches to meditation, all of which can be effective, and boast a number of mental and physical benefits.

Everybody is different. Finding which practice suits you is key. Some meditation is silent, some involves music, some involves deep thought, some only aim to clear the mind.

Meditation can be a great lead into getting a good night's deep sleep. Get an hour of meditation just before you go to bed, and it may help you rest better. Do not get discouraged if meditating is a challenge; for many of us, emptying our mind to this level can be very difficult at first. It's hard to stop our minds from racing about all that we have going on in our lives; however, this is key, and is exactly *why* meditation is so important.

We hold stress in our bodies. Our muscles, blood pressure, heart health, and hormonal balance can all be effected by our mental condition.

Our minds are quite powerful, and just like our bodies, giving them a regular break can help them run much more efficiently, and will allow them to do much more for us. The harder you push yourself, or the more pressure you put on yourself, or you find yourself under, the more meditation can do for you in the long run.

The physical benefits of meditation include increased serotonin production, which can boost mood and behavior. It can lower blood pressure, and reduce stress, increases energy and boosts the immune system.

The most positive effects of meditation can include increased focus, mental sharpness, mental energy, increased emotional stability, decreased anxiety, increases gray matter, brain volume, and cortical thickness which can promote self control, memory and attention span. Meditation has also been shown to boost your social activity.

As stated before, there are many different forms of meditation. If you find difficulty sitting still to meditate in the middle of the day, you can try going for a long walk in nature. Leave your smart phone behind, and try to become aware of your surroundings. Pay close attention to the small things. Stop and smell the roses, if you will.

Again, you should research and find the best meditation practice that suits *you*. For those who can't get enough sleep, try to sneak in 30-60 minutes of meditation either before bed, if you can't fall asleep, or later in the day if you need a break. It can make up for some deep rest that you may have missed.

Come into this experience with an open mind, and understand that when you accomplish meditation successfully, it can help you in so many ways, and you could reap the benefits of prolonged health as you age.

Meditation can vastly improve our quality of life, and requires very little of us in order to garner success. Stress is the cause of many ailments, and this is a great way to reduce and minimize all of the stress you may have in your life.

For athletes, meditation can be a great opportunity to focus on breathing. Control and awareness of breathing can help maximize power and endurance in athletics. You can learn to control your breath as well as your heart rate. This can be essential for getting the most out of your body when trying to perform.

You can also take this opportunity to become more self-aware. Meditation can help boost confidence, and self-esteem.

The wise are the ones who find ways to get better even when they aren't in the gym. The ones who make their overall, long-term, health a priority, will be well prepared later in life.

"All that we are is the result of what we have thought. The mind is everything. What you think, you become." - Buddha

SOAK UP THE RELAXATION

One of the absolute best ways that I have found to help my body to recover is the use of Epsom salt baths. As someone who has had back and neck problems since my teenage years, and a longtime combat athlete/wrestler, I felt extreme relief both literally and figuratively once I realized what detox baths can do for me.

Epsom salts have been around and used by many cultures for hundreds of years. Epsom Salt is actually not salt at all, it is a natural composition of minerals, which combine to create Magnesium Sulfate.

Magnesium sulfate can be absorbed through the skin and into the blood stream. Each component plays its own role and is valuable in its own right, but combined there are so many benefits to us. Primarily being detoxification, relaxation, reduced inflammation, and muscle recovery, as well as cleansing the skin through the use of its antifungal properties.

Epsom salt is an extremely cost efficient way to boost your recovery and improve body function, all while requiring minimal time (10-40 minutes). Epsom salt also has many household uses, and can be used to boost your personal organic garden, should you be raising one!

When purchasing, it's important to note that all Epsom salts are generally the same. Just make sure you are purchasing one that displays the initials U.S.P. which stands for United States Pharmacopeia, and that will let you know that its inspected and approved, and is the product it is advertised to be.

Magnesium Sulfates can also help with the mental recovery, which was discussed before. Deep relaxation achieved when taking an Epsom salt bath can be a fantastic time to practice your meditation, as well as provide preparation for deep sleep if done prior to bed. This can be especially beneficial when combined, as the great benefits of a good night of deep rest have been documented.

Epsom Salts will not just provide valuable minerals that you can absorb through your skin, but they also possess powerful detoxifying capabilities. Epsom salts draw actual salts and toxins from your skin, cleansing your system through a process referred to as reverse osmosis. This will also aid in weight loss, and will make you appear slimmer in its own right by reducing the sodium in your system and controlling the retention of water.

This process will cause you to sweat quite a bit, so it is important to replenish water and electrolytes sufficiently when utilizing Epsom salt baths. If done at the end of the night I usually add my second lemon squeeze to my water to maximize my detox. Each component of this compound can benefit you on its own.

Magnesium is a mineral found in the body in large amounts, however, many people unknowingly suffer from deficiencies in Magnesium, particularly women. This mineral plays a vital role in well over 300 important chemical reactions that take place within the human body, including promoting a higher absorption rate of calcium.

Magnesium can improve blood flow and oxygenate the blood, thus reducing inflammation as well as increasing energy and endurance, in addition to improving muscle function.   Athletes, or people who live active lives, that put a fair amount of strain on their bodies would likely see reductions in muscle tightness and injury from regular use of Epsom salt baths.

If you want to make sure you are getting enough magnesium in your diet, keep in mind that many green vegetables and natural foods are high in Magnesium. Generally, foods that are high in fiber tend to be rich in magnesium as well. For example, nuts, seeds, broccoli, and leafy green vegetables all boast high fiber as well as being rich in magnesium.

If a legitimate natural deficiency is confirmed, supplementation may be necessary. Coral calcium and

Magnesium are often paired together in supplementation, however, it can be supplemented individually in pill or cream form.

Sulfates promote healthy nervous tissue and support healthy joints, as well as cleansing and keeping the skin healthy. In synergy with Magnesium, Sulfates can be very beneficial for your health.

When taking an Epsom bath, you can receive benefits from 10-40 minutes of bath time, however 40 minutes is the suggested bath time. I suggest filling the bath to the appropriate height, and preferred temperature, add Epsom salt or bath salt mixture.

Start with 1-2 cups of Epsom salt. If your tub is larger, you can use more. Work your way up if need be, but initially the 1-2 cups should get the job done sufficiently, depending on your size. Then, swish the water around lightly until all of the salt mixture is dissolved into the water.

If your tub has an overflow drain that is too shallow, they do sell covers for the overflow drain. I suggest using caution if you use one, as the overflow drain is ultimately there for our protection.

The first twenty minutes of the bath is when our bodies go through the reverse osmosis process and the sodium and toxins are extracted through our skin. You will break your sweat and begin to relax.

The second twenty minutes is where we absorb the minerals into our bodies. If all you're looking for is a quick detox you can shorten your time, however, I usually try to get the full 40 minutes to maximize my benefits.

The water does not need to be hot, room temperature or slightly warm water will suffice. If you prefer hotter water, feel free to use the hottest that is comfortable for you.

If you want to get a heavier detox, and a heavier sweat, bath salts or sea salt can be added to the bath. I would start small and work your way up as this can make the bath more intense, and we want to get the full 40 minutes in, and remain relaxed rather than suffer through.

If you want to add natural products to moisturize your skin and keep it soft and smooth, then I would suggest Organic Powdered Milk. Oat bath products, baking soda, olive oil, and essential oils can also be added depending on preference. Coconut oil can be applied to skin and hair after bath for moisturizing and cell repair.

NATURAL HEALING

Essential Oils are extremely concentrated volatile oils, which are derived from plants and resins. What makes these oils "essential" is that these volatile oils contain the essence, or fragrance, of the plant itself.

Essential oils have been used for thousands of years to treat everything from skin conditions, to wounds, to mood, and even in some cultures disease and sickness. There are many different essential oils available today. They range in price, value, and beneficial importance.

Essential oils can be used in your baths, as many have great relaxing and recovery benefits; as massage oil; in making your own skin creams or lotions; in an oil diffuser for aromatherapy; and some can even be used in your diet.

There are more than 90 essential oils, most of which pair well together and can give you countless options to decide which combinations could be best for you. I strongly recommend that you do your research on Essential Oils as each one boasts its own specific benefits, and uses.

Not all Essential Oils are created equal, and this is a product where you typically get what you pay for. Good products can be highly expensive, however the more pure the product you're using, the less you need to use in order to reap the benefits. Many are in carrier oils such as jojoba oil. The more pure the product you can get, the better.

As I stated, there are over 90 essential oils available for use today. In this chapter I will go over some of my personal favorites and highlight some of the reasons that I use them. I suggest researching as much as you can and figure out which oils and brands suit you the best.

Lavender is probably the most common essential oil used because of its versatility, popular and pleasant aroma, and long list of benefits. Lavender is a natural disinfectant, promotes circulatory and respiratory health, offers pain relief, as well as a calming agent, and also helps to promote good deep sleep. Lavender can be used in baths, topical lotions, and aromatherapy.

Eucalyptus is great for muscles. It has anti-inflammatory and pain relief properties. Eucalyptus is also great for relieving chest congestion and treating the common cold as it stimulates the immune system. Eucalyptus is great in baths and skin creams, especially for aches and pains. It can also be used in aromatherapy.

Frankincense has serious anti aging properties and can do wonders for your skin and over all health. Frankincense has always been one of the most valuable essential oils, thus why it is also one of the most expensive, and also one that you should use the most caution when purchasing. You will want to spend the extra money to be assured you're getting a high quality product on this one. Because of the cost, I typically only use this one in a homemade skin cream. I do not add it to my baths. If you can afford to do so, it will work great in a bath as it has a wonderful scent

Myrrh has been used for thousands of years. Ancient Egyptians used Myrrh to embalm their pharaohs. It has fantastic anti-inflammatory and antioxidant properties. Myrrh can positively affect mood and hormone production in your body. Myrrh goes great in baths or skin creams, and can be used for aromatherapy.

Lemongrass can reduce pain in muscles, joints, and headaches. It has been shown to boost immune system, as well as confidence and self esteem. Lemongrass is great for baths as it has a great scent and isn't too expensive. In terms of value, it's a must.

Tea Tree Oil is fantastic for topical use on infections and wounds. It is great in baths to help treat sickness and the Bronchial congestion. Tea Tree Oil has balsamic properties, which promote general health by promoting the absorption of nutrients from the food we eat into our bodies as well as protect us against general disease.

Grapefruit oil boasts a wonderful scent, making it great for baths and skin creams, as well as aromatherapy. It has been used to treat migraine headaches, and is packed full of antioxidants. Grapefruit is a natural anti-depressant and a great natural stimulant. It has many benefits for your body and your mind. Grapefruit oil is a staple in my baths.

Peppermint oil has been known to have positive affects on digestion, respiratory, and liver health. Peppermint has been studied on its abilities to improve mental sharpness and focus. Peppermint is one of the few that goes well in food, as well as topical applications and aromatherapy.

Sandalwood is highly beneficial and is very diverse as an essential oil. It boasts antiseptic, anti-inflammatory, calming, and memory boosting properties. Quality is the concern with Sandalwood, as Indian Sandalwood is considered the best, but is also the most rare. Most Sandalwood products are made of Australian sandalwood, which is not as beneficial.

Lemon oil, not to be confused with lemongrass oil, is another beneficial citrus essential oil. Lemons are an amazing super-food and can provide us many benefits. Lemon oil is great for our skin, and immune support. It can be very calming and stress relieving in a bath or in aromatherapy. It has been used to treat insomnia and anxiety.

Oil of oregano is a great natural probiotic. It can reduce the amount of bad bacteria in your stomach and help support your immune system and help fight off sicknesses. It is normally taken orally or used topically on skin.

Coconut oil isn't really an Essential Oil, however it is simply too powerful to leave out. Coconut oil is great for repairing damaged hair and for moisturizing skin. When used in food it can provide some of the cleanest energy to our diets possible. Coconut oil can improve thyroid function and promotes proper insulin use in the body. Coconut oil is extremely healthy and can be very beneficial when used as a staple in weight loss and boosting athletic performance.

BODY MAINTENANCE

Chiropractic and physical therapy can be easy to skip. They can also go a long way towards making you feel better, and if you're active, it will certainly help you perform better.

It is important that we are always paying close attention to our bodies. If there are minor mechanical issue in our bodies, our minds will subliminally make changes in order for us to move without pain. We must be proactive and not always wait for the pain. It's best to avoid injuries rather than treat them as they come.

Seeing a chiropractor or a physical therapist occasionally, or regularly for some, can keep us on the right track and can stop the majority of our issues before they start. This can reduce our inflammation over time, which is definitely going to contribute to our long term health, and conserve energy that may have been wasted.

Foam rollers and massage balls can do wonders for those of us who are highly active, or have stiffness or soreness in our muscles. It's a great way to loosen muscles and work out lactic acid.

I use both a regular foam roller and a deep tissue roller. The deep tissue roller can be a little painful at first, but after a while you get used to it and it even starts to feel good. Foam rolling pairs well with stretching and massage therapy, and are wonderful pre and post workout recovery tools. In massaging the muscles, foam rollers help keep you in proper alignment and can help prevent serious injury when used regularly.

Massage balls are great if you have a stubborn sore muscle or if you are particularly stiff after a workout or a long day of work. Sit or lay with the ball underneath you on the targeted area, no rolling or movement is necessarily needed. Get good pressure and hold for a couple of minutes, let off the pressure and then stretch the specific muscle group. Repeat cycle 2-3 times or until targeted area has loosened.

Massage Therapy is one of the most commonly utilized tools of recovery. It is great for working out sore muscles and joints. Massage therapy pairs great with chiropractic adjustments for those who use a chiropractor. Massage therapy can help the adjustments take hold.

Massage therapy can also help by releasing the fascia between the skin and muscles, which can sometimes become tangled and knotted causing muscle pain and tension.

Massages reduce anxiety and depression, and can also be a great way for people to relieve general stress, may it be from personal or work life. We hold stress in our muscles, and getting a massage you can literally get that stress worked out of you.

Massage therapy improves circulation and range of motion, which is not only important for avoiding or recovering from injury, but also very important for keeping us healthy and active into an advanced age. As always, our goal is to maintain optimum long-term health.

When getting a massage, it is an opportunity to get in some meditation and take advantage of the relaxed state you will be in and the endorphins you will be releasing into your system.

Make sure to drink plenty of water before and after your massage. Deep tissue, in particular will release toxins that have built up in your muscles into your system to be flushed out. If you are dehydrated, some may remain in your system and make you sick.

Infrared saunas are one of my favorite devices to use for general muscle relaxation and to get a detoxifying sweat.

Infrared saunas differ from traditional saunas in that they do not heat the air. They actually heat your body, specifically. These saunas use infrared rays, which are invisible rays naturally emitted by the sun.

Infrared rays are the healthiest of those emitted by the sun; they penetrate deep into our skin, helping rid our body of accumulated toxins.

The sweat that occurs in the infrared sauna contains 17% toxins as opposed to 3% in a traditional sauna. Specifically, the toxins released by an infrared sauna are toxic metals that can build up in our system and be harmful to our health.

Infrared rays cause the water molecules in our bodies to vibrate and break down. This process causes the release of certain toxins.

Infrared saunas will cause you to sweat, however, you won't be subjected to the nearly unbearable temperatures of a traditional sauna. Infrared saunas typically run anywhere between 110-150 degrees Fahrenheit. Optimal temperature is usually between 110-130 degrees.

Studies show that it is possible to burn up to 700 calories in an infrared sauna session. Infrared sauna increases circulation, thus increasing metabolism and burning fat at a faster rate.

Infrared saunas heat our tissue, which enhances the metabolic process, enhancing cellular energy production and causing infections to heal faster. Damaged and diseased cells are weaker than healthy cells and tolerate heat poorly.

These saunas have been used to treat tendonitis, heart disease, hypertension, and osteoporosis, as well as helping to fight the common cold.

When using a sauna it is important to replenish the water and electrolytes that you will be losing through your sweat. It's best to use a sauna while wearing as little clothing as is comfortable as to not block the infrared rays.

Sauna temperature should be between 110-130 degrees Fahrenheit. Remain in infrared sauna for about 30-40 minutes per use or as long as is comfortable and safe.

One of the oldest forms of treating injuries and reducing inflammation is with the use of cryo-therapy. Cryo-therapy, for me, consists of three things. Cryo-sauana, Ice massage, and ice baths.

Ice massage or the use of ice packs is very common for treating pain, particularly with the use of athletic injuries, arthritis, and muscle soreness.

Typically, ice is used to treat acute injuries, or injuries that occur suddenly. It can also be used to treat some chronic injuries, which occur more due to overuse and over long periods of time. Generally, if inflammation is suspected, ice can be used to treat. If using an ice pack, rest pack on specific area of inflammation for 10 minutes, then rest for 5 minutes. Repeat this process three times, two to three times per day.

If using ice cups for an ice massage, you will massage area with an ice cup for 5 minutes and then rest for five minutes. Repeat the process two to three times per day.

To make an ice cup, fill a paper Dixie cup with water and freeze. Once frozen, tear the rim of the cup down so that the ice is exposed, use this to press down as firmly as possible without pain and massage gently. If massaging a larger area, use broad strokes.

Ice cups can penetrate a little deeper into your muscle than a regular ice pack but can be a little bit painful at first depending on the extent of your soreness.

If treating an injury, try to combine your ice routine with good compression therapy, which constricts and pressures the localized area and helps physically move toxins and inflammation out of the muscles and soft tissues.

In some cases, when treating an injury, heat is actually more appropriate. Chronic injuries tend to require more heat, particularly those involving joints and tendons. If an acute injury occurs, ice is usually needed first, however, after the inflammation is believed to have gone down, heat can help to bring blood flow to the area and remove toxins and lactic acid.

Ice baths have been used for a very long time, however they have really gained increased popularity in more recent years. They are typically used after strenuous activity or workouts. Sometimes they are used to treat injury.

Ice baths are when someone submerges into a tub filled with cold water ranging in temperature between 55- 65 degrees Fahrenheit, for a specific amount of time in an effort to aid in their recovery, and reduce pain and swelling.

The time increments of an ice bath can vary, as

there are many differing opinions on the topic. Some believe two minute increments, repeated ten times is a superior method, however others believe one 10-15 minute shot is better.

I personally have always taken ice baths in one shot ranging from 5-10 minutes at about 55-60 degrees Fahrenheit. This has always been sufficient for me, but can vary from person to person. If I don't take one for a while I'll go for about 6 minutes at 60 degrees. If I am taking them more regularly then I will intensify the treatment as I go.

Be very careful, do not take ice baths alone, and start off very slowly. Start with 2-3 minutes at 60-65 degrees and work your way down in temperature and/or longer time. DO NOT exceed 12 minutes ever, and do not attempt to go the full 12 minutes initially. It will take you a while to build up to that amount of time. Remember that moving water is colder than the temperature reads. It may help to wear protective gear around genitals and feet.

Some like to follow up their ice bath with either a hot shower, or a shower/bath with room temperature water depending on preference, however I would recommend getting out and warming up for a few minutes with a blanket first to give your body the time to warm a little more slowly. This will reduce the shock put on your body when going from extreme cold directly to extreme hot. You can even take it a step further and get a massage or foam-roll afterwards.

Cryo-sauna or cryo-chamber technology is the

newest rave in the recovery market. It is essentially the same concept as an ice bath, however, it is much more high tech and efficient.

Cryosaunas mix liquid nitrogen vapors with fresh air to create insanely cold temperatures. Cryo-sauanas reach temperatures in the range of -255 degrees Fahrenheit (-160 Celsius.)

These extreme temperatures lower our outer skin temperature to an astounding 40-50 degrees Fahrenheit. This causes our body to go into survival mode, and it begins to pull all of the blood to the inner core in an attempt to save our vital organs and sacrifice our limbs. After you emerge, your body realizes it is going to survive and moves the blood back out to the extremities.

This process creates a massive rush of endorphins and an instant increase in energy and mental focus. The major shift of blood through our bodies does wonders for reducing inflammation, and carrying out unwanted toxins and built up scar tissue in certain areas of the body.

While everything that we are learning from studies thus far has been extremely positive for Cryo-Sauna technology, it is still quite new and should be used in moderation. I would recommend using once per week to once per month depending on needs, or use as inflammation presents itself. I prefer to use this as preventative care for myself as muscle tightness often leads to larger injuries.

All of these methods, used on their own, or in conjunction, are essential in the continued care and optimization of your health and recovery process. I hope that this guide inspires you to expand your education on self-care and to create your own personal optimization plan. Thank you for taking the time to learn about how I embrace The Anti-Grind.